Islamic NLP: The Art of Communicating with God and Yourself

This book combines the principles of Neuro-Linguistic Programming (NLP) with Islamic spirituality. It offers a unique approach to personal development and self-improvement by showing readers how to use NLP techniques to enhance their communication with Allah (God) and better understand themselves.

The book discusses how the power of language can impact our thoughts, emotions, and behaviors, and how it can be used to create positive change in our lives. It explains how NLP techniques can be used to overcome limiting beliefs, negative self-talk, and unproductive behaviors, and how they can help us develop a more positive and empowering mindset.

The book also explores the Islamic perspective on personal development, emphasizing the importance of connecting with Allah and developing a strong relationship with Him. It offers practical guidance on how to use NLP techniques to strengthen one's faith, overcome spiritual challenges, and cultivate a more meaningful relationship with Allah.

"Islamic NLP: The Art of Communicating with God and Yourself" is a comprehensive guide that offers a new perspective on personal development and spiritual growth. It is an ideal resource for anyone looking to enhance their communication with Allah, deepen their understanding of themselves, and achieve their full potential.

Contents

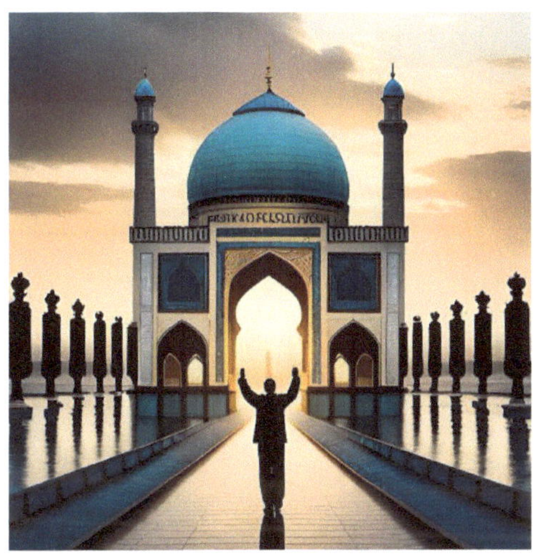

Introduction

Welcome to 'Islamic NLP: The Art of Communicating with God and Yourself.' This book is designed to help you understand how NLP techniques can be used to enhance your communication with Allah and deepen your understanding of yourself. Through the book, you'll learn how language impacts our thoughts, emotions, and behaviors, and how NLP techniques can be used to create positive change in your life. You'll also discover the Islamic perspective on personal development and spirituality, and how the combination of NLP and Islamic principles can help you achieve your full potential. In the following chapters, we'll explore the power of language, basic principles of NLP, and how NLP can be applied to various aspects of your life. By the end of the book, you'll have a practical understanding of how NLP and Islamic spirituality can help you connect with Allah and achieve personal growth."

Chapter 1- The Power of Language

It is in-depth exploration of the importance of language in our lives. The 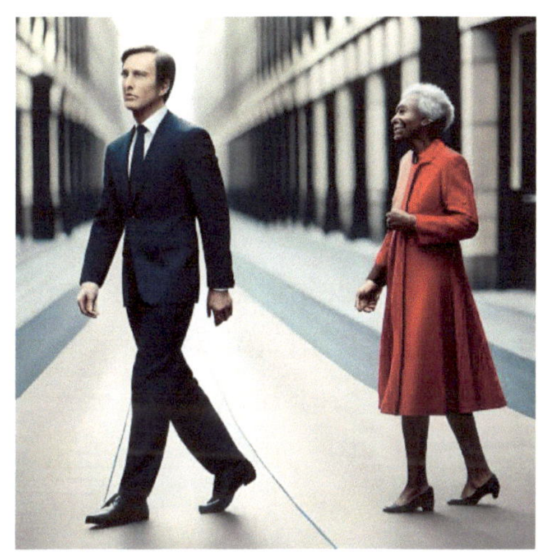 chapter is divided into three sections, each of which explores a different aspect of language: the science of language, the language of the self, and the language of spirituality.

How language impacts our thoughts, emotions, and behaviors

NLP is based on the idea that language and communication play a key role in shaping our thoughts, behaviors, and experiences. Therefore, understanding the science of language is crucial to understanding how NLP works.

One aspect of the Science of Language that is particularly relevant to NLP is the concept of "meta-modeling." Meta-modeling involves analyzing and understanding the structure of language and how it shapes our perception of reality. By understanding the underlying structure of language, NLP practitioners can identify patterns and beliefs that may be limiting or problematic, and work to change them.

Another important aspect of the Science of Language in NLP is the use of language patterns and techniques to achieve specific outcomes. For example, NLP practitioners may use "anchoring" techniques to associate positive emotions with a particular word or gesture, or use "reframing" techniques to shift the meaning of a negative experience to a more positive one. These techniques are based on an understanding of how language and communication can be used to influence and shape our thoughts and behaviors.

Overall, the Science of Language is an essential component of NLP, as it provides the theoretical foundation for many of the techniques and tools used in NLP practice. By understanding the science of language and how it shapes our thoughts and experiences, NLP practitioners can work to create positive change in themselves and others.

The relationship between language and personal development

"**The Language of the Self**" is equally important aspect of Neuro-Linguistic Programming (NLP). NLP recognizes that the language we use to describe ourselves and our experiences has a powerful impact on our thoughts, feelings, and behaviors. Therefore, understanding the language of the self is crucial to understanding how NLP works.

One aspect of the language of the self that is particularly relevant to NLP is the concept of "self-talk." Self-talk refers to the internal dialogue we have with ourselves, and the way in which we describe our experiences and beliefs. For example, someone with a negative self-talk pattern may describe themselves as "not good enough" or "always failing," while someone with a positive self-talk pattern may describe themselves as "capable" or "successful." By becoming aware of our self-talk patterns, we can begin to identify and change limiting beliefs and patterns that may be holding us back.

Another important aspect of the language of the self in NLP is the use of "self-reflexive" language. This involves using language to create a sense of distance between ourselves and our experiences, allowing us to observe and analyze them more objectively. For example, instead of saying "I am angry," we might say "I notice that I am feeling anger." This subtle shift in language can help us to become more aware of our emotions and thought patterns, and to make more conscious choices about how we respond to them.

Overall, the language of the self is a critical component of NLP, as it provides a powerful tool for self-awareness and personal growth. By becoming more mindful of our self-talk patterns and using self-reflexive language, we can begin to identify and change limiting beliefs and patterns, and create more positive and empowering experiences for ourselves.

The role of language in Islamic spirituality

Neuro-Linguistic Programming (NLP) and its intersection with Islam. Islam places a great emphasis on spiritual development, and language plays a key role in this process. Therefore, understanding the language of spirituality is crucial to understanding how NLP and Islam can be used together to promote personal growth and well-being.

One aspect of the language of spirituality that is particularly relevant to NLP and Islam is the concept of "remembrance" or "dhikr." Dhikr is a practice in Islam that involves repeating the names of Allah, reciting Quranic verses, and reflecting on the attributes of Allah. NLP practitioners can use similar techniques to cultivate a positive and empowering mindset, such as repeating affirmations or visualizing positive outcomes.

Another important aspect of the language of spirituality in NLP and Islam is the use of metaphor and symbolism to convey spiritual concepts. In Islam, the Quran is full of metaphors and symbols that are used to illustrate spiritual truths and convey deeper meanings. Similarly, NLP practitioners can use metaphor and symbolism to help clients understand and internalize complex concepts and ideas.

Overall, the language of spirituality is a critical component of NLP and its intersection with Islam, as it provides a powerful tool for personal and spiritual growth. By understanding and using the language of spirituality in NLP practice, practitioners can help clients to connect with their inner selves and tap into their spiritual potential, leading to a deeper sense of fulfillment and well-being.

Chapter 2: Understanding NLP

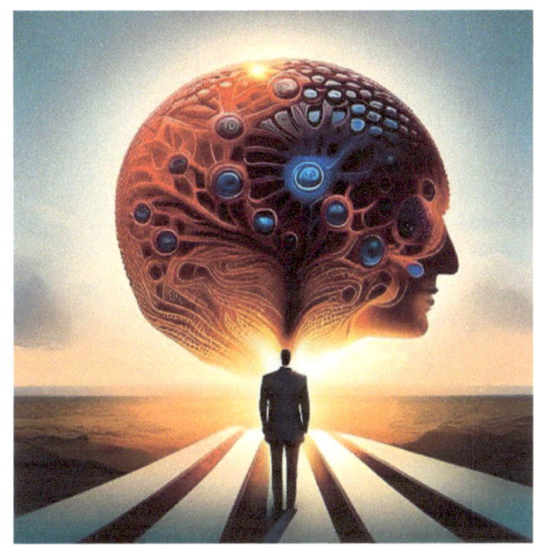

Neuro-Linguistic Programming (NLP) is a method of communication and personal development that focuses on the relationship between thoughts, language, and behavior. Here are some examples of how NLP works in practice:

Anchoring: Anchoring is a technique used in NLP to create a connection between a certain trigger (such as a sound or a word) and a desired emotional state. For example, a person might use anchoring to feel confident and calm before a public speaking event. They would recall a time when they felt confident and calm, and then associate that feeling with a specific trigger, such as pressing their thumb and forefinger together. Then, before the public speaking event, they would press their thumb and forefinger together to anchor that feeling of confidence and calm.

Reframing: Reframing is a technique used in NLP to change the way a person perceives a situation by putting it in a different context. For example, a person who is nervous about a job interview might reframe the situation by thinking of it as an opportunity to showcase their skills and experience. By changing the way they perceive the situation, they can change the way they feel about it and approach it with more confidence.

Modeling: Modeling is a technique used in NLP to learn from someone who is already successful in a particular area. For example, a salesperson might model the communication style and techniques of a top-performing salesperson in their company in order to improve their own sales performance.

Sensory acuity: Sensory acuity is a technique used in NLP to improve the ability to read nonverbal cues and body language. By becoming more attuned to subtle changes in a person's facial expressions, posture, and tone of voice, a person can gain a better understanding of their emotions and thoughts.

Meta-programs: Meta-programs are patterns of thought and behavior that influence the way a person processes information and makes decisions. For example, a person might have a meta-program of "toward" motivation, meaning they are more motivated by the prospect of achieving a positive outcome than by the fear of avoiding a negative outcome. By understanding their meta-programs, a person can gain insights into their own behavior and make more conscious choices about how they respond to different situations.

These are just a few examples of how NLP works in practice. Overall, NLP provides a wide range of tools and techniques that can help individuals to communicate more effectively, understand their own behavior and thought patterns, and achieve their personal and professional goals.

Basic principles of NLP

If you understand this section, it gives an ease to understand the broader picture of NLP.

The Map is Not the Territory: This principle acknowledges that each person's perception of the world is subjective and unique. NLP practitioners believe that a person's experience of the world is filtered through their senses, memories, and beliefs. For example, imagine two people who attend the same concert. One person might describe it as "energetic and exciting" while another might describe it as "overwhelming and chaotic." Both descriptions are valid, but they reflect each person's unique experience of the concert.

Rapport: Rapport is the ability to establish a connection with another person and create a sense of mutual understanding and trust. NLP practitioners believe that establishing rapport is essential for effective communication and building strong relationships. For example, a salesperson might use mirroring techniques to match the body language and tone of voice of their potential customer in order to establish rapport and build trust.

Outcome-Oriented: NLP practitioners believe that defining clear and specific outcomes is essential for achieving success. By setting clear goals and outcomes, individuals can focus their attention and resources on achieving them. For example, a person might set a goal to run a marathon within six months. By defining this outcome, they can create a plan for training, establish metrics for tracking their progress, and stay motivated throughout the process.

Feedback: NLP practitioners believe that feedback is essential for learning and growth. By seeking and responding to feedback, individuals can identify areas for improvement and adjust their behavior and strategies accordingly. For example, a manager might provide feedback to an employee on their presentation skills in order to help them improve and achieve better results.

State Management: NLP practitioners believe that a person's emotional state can significantly impact their behavior and ability to achieve their goals. By learning to manage their emotional states, individuals can improve their performance and decision-making. For example, a person might use breathing techniques or visualization exercises to manage their anxiety before a job interview.

Sensory Acuity: NLP practitioners believe that developing sensory acuity - the ability to observe and interpret nonverbal cues - is essential for effective communication. By paying attention to subtle changes in a person's body language, tone of voice, and facial expressions, individuals can gain insight into their thoughts and emotions. For example, a teacher might notice that a student is avoiding eye contact and fidgeting during class, indicating that they might be struggling with a particular subject or feeling anxious.

Behavioral Flexibility: NLP practitioners believe that having behavioral flexibility - the ability to adapt to different situations and communication styles - is essential for effective communication and problem-solving. By being open to different perspectives and approaches, individuals can find creative solutions to challenges. For example, a manager might need to adapt their leadership style to motivate a team of employees with different personalities and work styles.

Chunking: NLP practitioners believe that chunking - breaking down information into smaller, more manageable pieces - can help individuals better understand and process complex information. By grouping related pieces of information together, individuals can identify patterns and connections. For example, a student might use chunking to better understand a difficult chapter in a textbook by breaking it down into smaller sections and identifying key concepts.

Anchoring: NLP practitioners believe that anchoring - associating a particular state or emotion with a specific trigger - can be used to control and manage emotions. By creating positive anchors, individuals can access positive emotional states when needed. For example, a person might create a physical anchor - such as squeezing their fist - to trigger a positive emotional state, such as confidence, before a public speaking engagement.

By applying these principles, individuals can improve their communication skills, enhance their personal and professional relationships, and achieve their goals.

NLP techniques for personal development

NLP techniques can be effective for personal development by helping individuals identify and overcome limiting beliefs and negative thought patterns. Here are some examples of NLP techniques that can be used for personal development:

Anchoring: Anchoring is a technique used to associate a positive emotional state with a specific trigger, such as a touch, sound, or word.

For example, an individual can anchor a feeling of confidence by associating it with a particular gesture, like making a fist. Whenever they feel they need an extra boost of confidence, they can trigger this state by performing the same gesture.

Reframing: Reframing involves changing the way a person perceives a situation by looking at it from a different perspective. For example, if an individual feels like they are failing at a particular task, a therapist using NLP might help them reframe their thinking by asking them to identify the areas where they are succeeding in that same task.

Swish pattern: The Swish pattern is a technique used to replace negative thoughts or behaviors with positive ones. For example, if someone has a habit of procrastinating, they can use the Swish pattern to replace the thought of procrastinating with the thought of starting the task immediately.

Timeline therapy: Timeline therapy is a technique used to help individuals overcome negative emotions and limiting beliefs from past experiences. By revisiting past memories, individuals can identify and release negative emotions and limiting beliefs that are holding them back.

Visualizing: Visualizing is a technique used to create a mental image of a desired outcome. For example, an athlete might use visualization to imagine themselves performing at their best during a competition. This technique can help individuals develop the confidence and motivation they need to achieve their goals.

Meta-modeling: Meta-modeling is a technique used to identify and challenge limiting beliefs and assumptions. A therapist might use meta-modeling to ask a client to clarify their language, and to help them identify when they are making assumptions that may not be true.

By working with a trained NLP practitioner or therapist, individuals can learn how to identify and overcome negative thought patterns and behaviors and develop new ways of thinking and behaving that support their personal growth and development.

The benefits of using NLP in Islamic spirituality

The use of NLP in Islamic spirituality can offer several benefits to individuals looking to deepen their understanding and practice of their faith. Here are some examples:

Developing a deeper connection with Allah: NLP techniques can help individuals develop a stronger connection with Allah and enhance their spiritual experiences. For example, using visualization techniques can help individuals create a mental image of Allah and connect with His presence.

Overcoming limiting beliefs: NLP techniques can be effective in identifying and overcoming limiting beliefs that may be holding individuals back from fully embracing their faith. For example, a person who has negative beliefs about themselves or their ability to follow Islamic principles can use NLP techniques to reframe their thinking and develop more positive beliefs.

Improving communication with others: NLP techniques can improve communication skills, which is an essential part of Islamic spirituality. Effective communication with others can help individuals build stronger relationships, deepen their understanding of others, and enhance their ability to spread the message of Islam.

Managing emotions: NLP techniques can help individuals manage their emotions and reduce negative emotions such as anger, frustration, and fear. This can help individuals remain calm and focused during times of stress or difficult situations, which is important in Islamic spirituality.

Setting and achieving goals: NLP techniques can help individuals set and achieve goals that are aligned with their Islamic values. For example, by using anchoring techniques, individuals can associate positive emotions with specific Islamic practices, such as praying, fasting, or giving to charity, which can help them stay motivated and committed to these practices.

Enhancing self-awareness: NLP techniques can help individuals become more self-aware, which is essential in Islamic spirituality. By identifying and understanding their thoughts, feelings, and behaviors, individuals can develop a deeper understanding of themselves and their relationship with Allah.

Overall, the use of NLP in Islamic spirituality can offer many benefits to individuals looking to enhance their spiritual experiences, deepen their connection with Allah, and improve their personal growth and development.

Chapter 3: Overcoming Limiting Beliefs

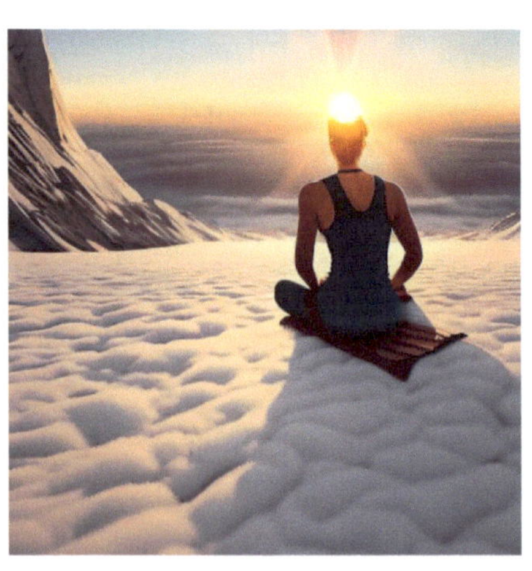

Chapter 3 of "Islamic NLP: The Art of Communicating with God and Yourself" focuses on the topic of overcoming limiting beliefs, which are beliefs that hold us back from achieving our goals and realizing our full potential. These beliefs are often deeply ingrained in our minds and can be challenging to identify and overcome. However, the techniques of NLP can help individuals overcome these beliefs and live a more fulfilling life.

NLP techniques for overcoming limiting beliefs

One technique that can be used to overcome limiting beliefs is the "reimprinting" technique. This technique involves revisiting a past experience that may have contributed to the formation of a limiting belief and then changing the way we think about that experience. The steps to apply the reimprinting technique are as follows:

1. Identify the limiting belief: The first step is to identify the limiting belief that you want to work on. This could be a belief related to your career, relationships, or personal growth.

2. Identify the root cause: The next step is to identify the root cause of the limiting belief. This could be a past experience or event that contributed to the formation of the belief.

3. Reimprint the experience: Once you have identified the root cause, you can reimprint the experience by changing the way you think about it. For example, if the limiting belief is "I am not good enough," you can reimprint the experience by reframing it to "I am always learning and growing."

Another technique that can be used to overcome limiting beliefs is called "anchoring." Anchoring involves associating a particular feeling or emotion with a specific action or thought. For example, if you have a limiting belief about your ability to succeed in your career, you can anchor a positive emotion to the thought of success. The steps to apply the anchoring technique are as follows:

1. Identify the limiting belief: The first step is to identify the limiting belief that you want

to work on. This could be a belief related to your career, relationships, or personal growth.

2. Identify the positive emotion: The next step is to identify a positive emotion that you want to associate with the thought of success. This could be a feeling of confidence, happiness, or excitement.

3. Create an anchor: Once you have identified the positive emotion, you can create an anchor by associating it with a physical action, such as touching your thumb and forefinger together.

4. Practice the anchor: You can practice the anchor by repeatedly associating the physical action with the positive emotion. Over time, the physical action will become associated with the positive emotion, and

you can use it to counteract the limiting belief.

The Islamic perspective on overcoming limiting beliefs

In Islamic spirituality, limiting beliefs can often be related to one's faith and connection with God. By using NLP techniques, individuals can overcome these limiting beliefs and strengthen their relationship with God. Practical steps for applying NLP techniques in Islamic spirituality include:

1. Identifying limiting beliefs related to one's faith, such as the belief that one is not good enough to fully embrace their faith.

2. Using the reimprinting technique to reframe the limiting belief in a positive light, such as "I am always growing in my faith."

3. Anchoring positive emotions, such as joy
   and fulfillment, to religious practices to
   counteract limiting beliefs.

Overall, the techniques outlined in Chapter 3 can be applied to many different areas of life, including relationships, career, and personal growth, as well as Islamic spirituality. By overcoming limiting beliefs, individuals can live a more fulfilling life and strengthen their connection with God.

Chapter 4: Developing a Positive Mindset

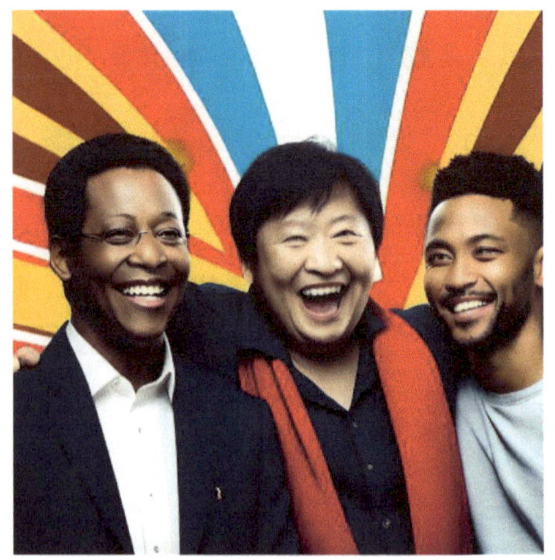

A positive mindset is crucial for personal growth and success in all areas of life. This chapter explores the concept of developing a positive mindset using NLP techniques that can be applied in Islamic spirituality.

How our mindset affects our lives

The first step in developing a positive mindset is to identify and replace negative self-talk with positive affirmations. Negative self-talk can lead to feelings of self-doubt, low self-esteem, and anxiety. On the other hand, positive affirmations can help to build confidence, resilience, and a sense of inner peace. For example, instead of saying "I can't do this," you can say "I am capable and strong enough to face any challenge."

NLP techniques for developing a positive mindset

Another NLP technique for developing a positive mindset is visualization. Visualization involves creating a mental image of the desired outcome and experiencing the emotions and sensations associated with that outcome. For example, if you want to improve your performance in a particular task, you can visualize yourself performing that task with confidence and ease.

Anchoring is another powerful NLP technique that can help in developing a positive mindset. Anchoring involves associating a particular emotional state with a physical trigger such as touching your thumb and index finger together. This trigger can be used to recall the positive emotional state when needed, such as during moments of stress or anxiety.

The language we use is also important in developing a positive mindset. By changing the way we talk about ourselves and our experiences, we can shift our mindset from a negative to a positive one. For example, instead of saying "I failed," you can say "I learned from my mistakes and will do better next time."

One practical step for developing a positive mindset is to create a gratitude journal. This involves writing down three things you are grateful for every day, no matter how small they may seem. Focusing on the positive aspects of your life can help to shift your mindset towards positivity.

The Islamic perspective on positivity and gratitude

In Islamic spirituality, developing a positive mindset is also linked to having faith in Allah's plan and trusting in His mercy. By aligning our thoughts and actions with our faith, we can cultivate a positive mindset that is rooted in gratitude, humility, and contentment.

Chapter 5: Communication with Allah

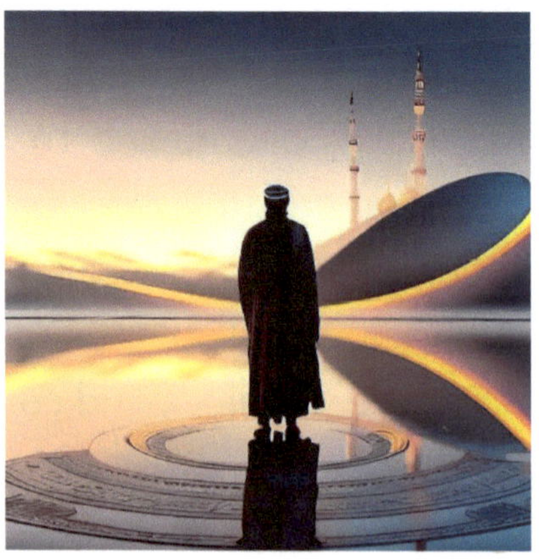

Effective communication is an essential component of any healthy relationship, including our relationship with Allah. In this chapter, we explore the concept of communication with Allah and how NLP techniques can be applied to enhance this communication.

The importance of communication with Allah in Islamic spirituality

Firstly, it is important to understand that communication with Allah is not a one-way street. Allah communicates with us through His divine guidance in the Quran and through the teachings of the Prophet Muhammad (peace be upon him). As Muslims, we communicate with Allah through various forms of worship, including prayer, supplication, and remembrance.

However, sometimes our communication with Allah can be hindered by various factors, such as distractions, negative thoughts, and doubts. NLP techniques can help us to overcome these obstacles and improve our communication with Allah.

NLP techniques for enhancing communication with Allah

One NLP technique that can enhance our communication with Allah is reframing. Reframing involves changing the way we view a situation or experience by shifting our focus to a more positive or empowering perspective. For example, if we are experiencing a difficult trial or hardship, we can reframe our thoughts by reminding ourselves that this is a test from Allah and that He has promised to never burden us with more than we can bear.

Another NLP technique that can be used for communication with Allah is anchoring. As mentioned earlier, anchoring involves associating a particular emotional state with a physical trigger. We can use this technique to anchor positive emotional states, such as gratitude or contentment, to our acts of worship. For example, we can touch our thumb and index finger together as we recite a particular supplication or verse from the Quran to anchor the positive emotions associated with that act of worship.

Visualization is another powerful NLP technique that can be applied to communication with Allah. We can visualize ourselves in a state of deep connection with Allah during our acts of worship, such as prayer or recitation of the Quran. We can also visualize ourselves receiving guidance and blessings from Allah in our daily lives.

Tips for developing a stronger relationship with Allah

The language we use in our communication with Allah is also important. By using positive and empowering language, we can enhance our connection with Allah and improve the quality of our communication. For example, instead of making demands in our supplications, we can express our needs and desires with humility and gratitude. We can also use positive affirmations to remind ourselves of Allah's mercy and blessings.

In Islamic spirituality, the concept of mindfulness is also closely related to communication with Allah. Mindfulness involves being fully present in the moment and aware of our thoughts and emotions. By practicing mindfulness during our acts of worship, we can enhance our connection with Allah and improve the quality of our communication.

One practical step for enhancing our communication with Allah is to set aside dedicated time for reflection and introspection. This can involve journaling, reciting the Quran, or simply taking a few moments to reflect on our thoughts and emotions. By regularly taking time to connect with Allah and reflect on our relationship with Him, we can deepen our communication and strengthen our faith.

In conclusion, communication with Allah is a vital component of our spiritual growth and development as Muslims. By applying NLP techniques, we can overcome obstacles that hinder our communication and enhance the quality of our connection with Allah. By striving to improve our communication with Allah, we can strengthen our faith, find inner peace, and ultimately, attain success in this life and the hereafter.

Chapter 6: Self-Discovery and Personal Growth

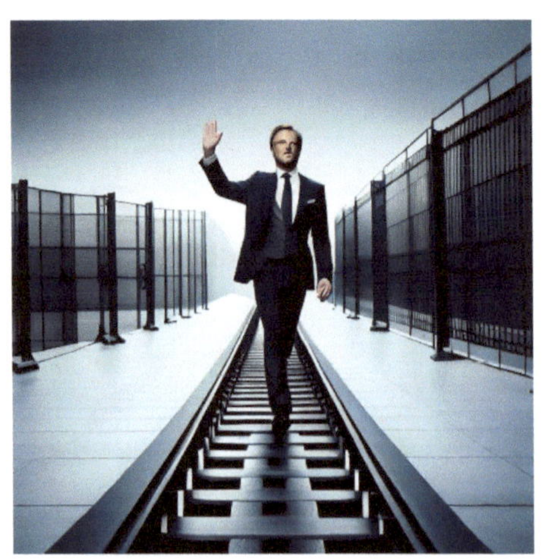

Self-discovery and personal growth are essential components of spiritual development in Islam. By discovering ourselves, we can understand our strengths and weaknesses, and use them to improve our lives and our relationship with Allah. Personal growth is a lifelong journey, and it involves continuous learning, self-awareness, and self-improvement.

Understanding yourself better through NLP

In this chapter, we will discuss how NLP can be used to facilitate self-discovery and personal growth in Islam. NLP techniques can help us explore our thoughts, beliefs, and values, and discover our true potential. Here are some examples of NLP techniques that can be used for self-discovery and personal growth:

NLP techniques for self-discovery and personal growth

Anchoring: Anchoring is a technique that can be used to create a positive association with a particular state of mind or emotion. For example, if you want to feel more confident during prayer, you can anchor that feeling by associating it with a physical gesture or a word. Whenever you perform that gesture or say that word, you will automatically feel more confident.

Reframing: Reframing is a technique that can be used to change the meaning of a particular situation or experience. For example, if you have a negative experience during prayer, you can reframe it by looking at it from a different perspective. You can focus on what you have learned from the experience, or how it has helped you grow spiritually.

Visualisation: Visualisation is a technique that can be used to create a mental image of a desired outcome or goal. For example, if you want to improve your relationship with Allah, you can visualise yourself having a deep and meaningful connection with Him. This can help you stay motivated and focused on your goal.

Self-talk: Self-talk is a technique that involves the use of positive affirmations and self-talk to improve your self-esteem and confidence. For example, you can repeat positive affirmations to yourself during prayer, such as "I am a good Muslim" or "I am grateful for the blessings in my life".

The Islamic perspective on self-awareness and personal growth

By using these and other NLP techniques, you can develop a deeper understanding of yourself, and discover new ways to grow and develop spiritually. Additionally, you can use these techniques to identify and overcome any limiting beliefs or negative thought patterns that may be holding you back. Through self-discovery and personal growth, you can become a better Muslim and strengthen your relationship with Allah.

Chapter 7: Applying NLP in Daily Life

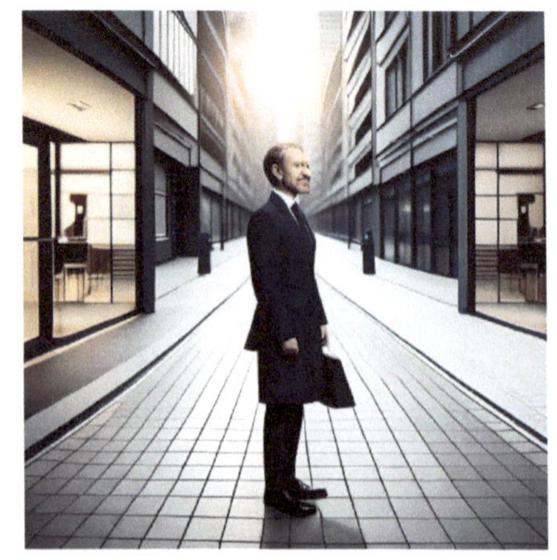

In this chapter, we will explore how NLP techniques can be applied in our daily lives to help us achieve our goals, communicate effectively, and improve our relationships with others.

Integrating NLP techniques into daily routines

Goal Setting:

One of the key principles of NLP is setting goals that are specific, measurable, achievable, relevant, and time-bound. This helps in achieving clarity of what you want to achieve and how to achieve it. For example, if you want to become more organized, your goal could be "I will organize my closet by the end of this week by donating clothes I haven't worn in the last year."

Mindful Communication:

NLP teaches us the importance of mindful communication. One technique is to use "I" statements instead of "you" statements. For example, instead of saying "You never listen to me," you can say, "I feel unheard when I try to communicate with you." This shift in language helps to take responsibility for your feelings and avoid putting the other person on the defensive.

Rapport Building:

NLP emphasizes the importance of building rapport with others. One way to build rapport is through mirroring and matching. This means matching the other person's tone of voice, body language, and breathing rate. This helps to create a sense of trust and empathy.

Anchoring:

Anchoring is a powerful NLP technique that can help us change our state of mind. For example, you can create an anchor by associating a positive emotion, such as joy or gratitude, with a physical action like tapping your chest or taking a deep breath. Whenever you want to access that positive emotion, you can use the physical anchor to trigger it.

Reframing:

NLP teaches us to reframe our negative experiences and thoughts in a positive light. For example, instead of saying "I can't do this," you can reframe it as "I haven't figured out how to do this yet." This helps to shift your mindset from one of defeat to one of possibility.

Time Management:

NLP techniques can also be used to improve time management skills. For example, you can use chunking to break down larger tasks into smaller, more manageable ones. You can also use visualization to help you prioritize your tasks and allocate your time effectively.

Overcoming Procrastination:

NLP can also help us overcome procrastination. One technique is to visualize the consequences of not completing a task. For example, if you're procrastinating on a work assignment, visualize the negative consequences of not completing it on time, such as missing a deadline or losing a client.

Managing Stress:

NLP techniques can also be used to manage stress. One technique is to use deep breathing exercises to calm your mind and body. You can also use visualization to imagine yourself in a calm and relaxing environment.

The Islamic perspective on practical applications of NLP

NLP, or Neuro-Linguistic Programming, is a set of techniques and principles that aim to help individuals achieve their goals and improve their lives by improving their communication and thought processes. While NLP is not explicitly tied to any particular religious or spiritual tradition, it can certainly be applied within an Islamic framework. From an Islamic perspective, the ultimate goal of any self-improvement or personal growth practice is to become closer to Allah and to live a life in accordance with His guidance.

One of the most important principles of NLP is the idea of taking responsibility for one's own thoughts and actions. In Islam, this principle is known as "taqwa," which means being conscious and aware of Allah in all aspects of one's life. By applying NLP techniques to cultivate greater awareness and control over our own thoughts and behaviors, we can strengthen our taqwa and become more aligned with Islamic values.

Another key aspect of NLP is the emphasis on positive thinking and visualization. In Islam, the concept of "tawakkul" refers to placing trust in Allah and having faith in His plan. By cultivating a positive mindset and visualizing positive outcomes, we can strengthen our tawakkul and develop a deeper sense of trust in Allah's plan for us.

NLP can also be applied in the context of interpersonal relationships, which are a crucial aspect of Islamic spirituality. By using NLP techniques to improve our communication and understanding of others, we can strengthen our relationships with family, friends, and community members, and create a more harmonious and supportive environment.

In addition, NLP can be applied in the context of personal growth and self-discovery. By using NLP techniques such as timeline therapy and reframing, we can gain a deeper understanding of our own thought patterns and beliefs, and work to overcome limiting beliefs and negative self-talk. This can help us to cultivate greater self-awareness and develop a stronger connection with Allah.

Overall, the Islamic perspective on practical applications of NLP emphasizes the importance of aligning our personal growth and self-improvement efforts with our faith and values. By using NLP techniques to become more conscious and aware of our thoughts and behaviors, and to develop a deeper sense of trust and connection with Allah, we can create a more fulfilling and purposeful life that is grounded in Islamic spirituality.

Conclusion

In conclusion, Neuro-Linguistic Programming (NLP) is a powerful tool that can be used in various aspects of life, including 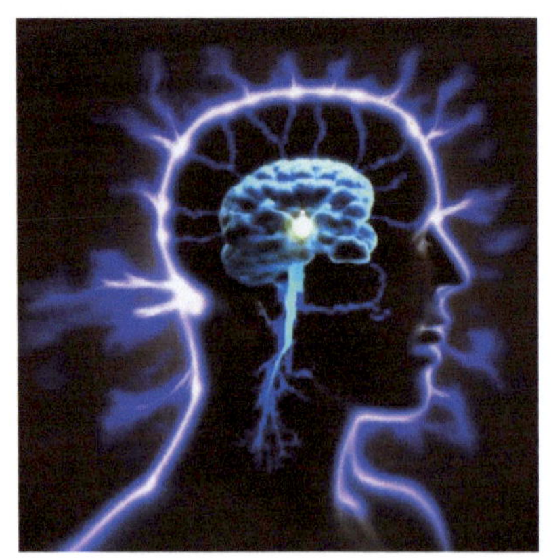 personal development, communication, and spiritual growth. Through the techniques and principles of NLP, individuals can learn to overcome limiting beliefs, develop a positive mindset, and communicate more effectively with themselves and others.

When it comes to Islamic spirituality, the application of NLP techniques can provide additional benefits, such as improving one's relationship with Allah, increasing self-awareness, and fostering personal growth. NLP principles are aligned with Islamic teachings on self-improvement, and can serve as a complementary tool to traditional Islamic practices such as meditation, prayer, and self-reflection.

By applying NLP techniques in daily life, individuals can experience tangible benefits, such as improved relationships, increased confidence, and better overall well-being. These techniques can be applied in various settings, including the workplace, personal relationships, and even in spiritual practices.

Overall, the principles of NLP and its practical applications can greatly enhance one's personal and spiritual development. By understanding and utilizing these techniques, individuals can overcome limitations, develop a positive mindset, and improve their communication skills, ultimately leading to a more fulfilling and purposeful life.

Summary of key points

- Neuro-Linguistic Programming (NLP) is a powerful tool that can be used in various aspects of life, including personal development, communication, and spiritual growth.
- NLP techniques can help individuals overcome limiting beliefs, develop a positive mindset, and communicate more effectively with themselves and others.
- The application of NLP techniques in Islamic spirituality can provide additional benefits, such as improving one's relationship with Allah, increasing self-awareness, and fostering personal growth.
- NLP principles are aligned with Islamic teachings on self-improvement and can complement traditional Islamic practices such as meditation, prayer, and self-reflection.
- By applying NLP techniques in daily life, individuals can experience tangible benefits such as improved relationships,

increased confidence, and better overall well-being.

- NLP can be applied in various settings, including the workplace, personal relationships, and even in spiritual practices.
- The principles of NLP and its practical applications can greatly enhance one's personal and spiritual development, leading to a more fulfilling and purposeful life.

Final thoughts on the benefits of combining NLP and Islamic spirituality

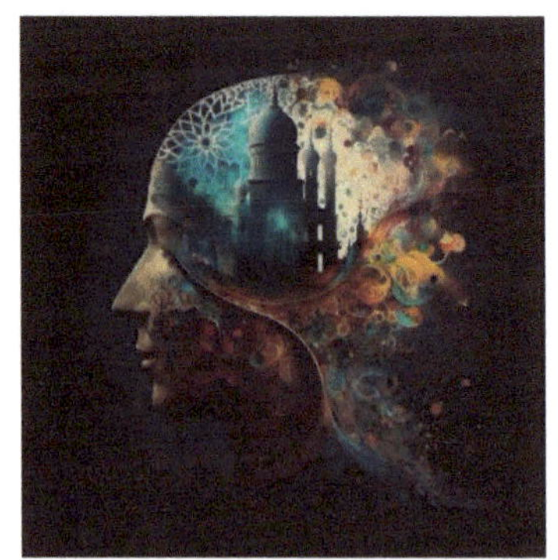

Combining NLP and Islamic spirituality can offer a multitude of benefits for individuals seeking personal and spiritual growth. By incorporating NLP techniques into their daily lives, Muslims can enhance their connection with Allah, deepen their understanding of themselves and others, and develop a positive mindset that is conducive to growth and success.

Furthermore, the principles of NLP are in line with Islamic teachings on self-improvement, such as self-awareness, self-reflection, and taking responsibility for one's actions. NLP can provide a practical framework for implementing these teachings and can help Muslims overcome obstacles that may be hindering their spiritual progress.

Overall, the integration of NLP and Islamic spirituality can lead to a more holistic approach to personal and spiritual growth, providing individuals with the tools and guidance they need to live a more fulfilling and purposeful life.

Sources

Some credible sources for more information on NLP and Islamic spirituality include books by Mobeen Vaid and "The Spiritual Practices of Rumi: Radical Techniques for Beholding the Divine" by Will Johnson. Additionally, reputable websites such as the International Association of NLP and Coaching can provide further insight and resources on the topics.

- Bandler, R., & Grinder, J. (1979). Frogs into princes: Neuro linguistic programming. Moab, UT: Real People Press.
- Dilts, R., Grinder, J., Bandler, R., & DeLozier, J. (1980). Neuro-Linguistic Programming: Volume I: The Study of the Structure of Subjective Experience. Cupertino, CA: Meta Publications.
- O'Connor, J., & Seymour, J. (1994). Introducing Neuro-Linguistic Programming: Psychological Skills for Understanding and Influencing People. London: HarperCollins.

- Andreas, S., & Andreas, C. (2009). NLP: The New Technology of Achievement. New York: HarperCollins.
- Hall, L., & Bodenhamer, B. (2012). The User's Manual for the Brain: The Complete Manual for Neuro-Linguistic Programming Practitioner Certification. Wales: Crown House Publishing.
- Grinder, M. (2011). Precision: A New Approach to Communication. London: Routledge.
- Sturt, D., & Palin, G. (2012). NLP Coaching: An Evidence-Based Approach for Coaches, Leaders and Individuals. London: Crown House Publishing.
- Zeig, J. K., & Lankton, S. R. (2014). The Handbook of Ericksonian Psychotherapy. Milton Park, Abingdon, Oxon: Routledge.
- Dilts, R., Delozier, J., & Bateson, G. (2001). The Encyclopedia of Systemic NLP and NLP New Coding. Scotts Valley, CA: NLP University Press.

Thank you

I owe a debt of gratitude to the incredible Mrs. Kanwal Rizvi, my NLP & Life Coach, for leading me on a transformative journey of self-discovery. I'm forever grateful for my parents and spouse, whose unwavering support has been a constant source of strength and motivation. Additionally, I must mention the exceptional NLP coaches Ms. Maria, Dr. Nabila & Mr. Ahsan, who went above and beyond to offer their guidance and support. Together, these individuals have opened up a whole new world of possibilities for me, and I can't thank them enough for their contribution to my personal growth and development.